Priority Setting Processes for Healthcare

in Oregon, USA; New Zealand; The Netherlands; Sweden; and the United Kingdom

Frank Honigsbaum
Senior Research Fellow
Health Services Management Centre
University of Birmingham

Dr Johann Calltorp
Professor
Health Services
Management Nordic School
of Public Health, Gothenburg

Chris Ham
Professor and Director
Health Services Management Centre
University of Birmingham

Dr Stefan Holmström
Director
Department of Community Medicine
Stockholm County Council

RADCLIFFE MEDICAL PRESS
Oxford and New York

©1995 Radcliffe Medical Press Ltd.
15 Kings Meadow, Ferry Hinksey Road, Oxford, OX2 0DP, UK

Radcliffe Medical Press, Inc
141 Fifth Avenue, New York, NY 10010, USA

British Library Cataloguing in Publication Data

A Catalogue record for this book is available from the British Library

ISBN 1 85775 033 0

Typeset by AMA Graphics Ltd., Preston
Printed and bound in Great Britain

Contents

Contents

Seminar Participants

The Netherlands: Wynand van de Ven, *Erasmus University, Rotterdam*

New Zealand Wendy Edgar, *Core Services Committee, Ministry of Health, Wellington*

Sweden: Christina Bolund, *Oncology Department, Karolinka Hospital*
Johann Calltorp, *Health Services Management, Nordic School of Public Health*
Lars-Olof Eklund, *Department of Community Medicine, Huddinge Hospital*
Mary Frank, *Vasterbotten County Council*
Hans Gilljam, *Department of Chest Medicine, Huddinge Hospital*
Stefan Holmström, *Department of Community Medicine, Huddinge Hospital*
Bengt Lundgren, *Department of Radiology, Gavleborg County Council*

Anders Paperin, *Economist, Primary Care*
Olle Saemund, *Department of
  Anaesthetics, Udedevalla Hospital*
Margareta Soderberg, *Department of
  Community Medicine, Huddinge
  Hospital*
Jan Thorling, *Department of
  Orthopaedic Surgery, Falu Hospital*
Sonia Wallin, *Oncology Department,
  Karolinska Hospital*
Helena Westerberg, *Oncology
  Department, Karolinska Hospital*

United Kingdom: Geoffrey Carroll, *North Essex District
  Health Authority*
Chris Ham, *University of Birmingham*
Sandy Hogg, *Oxfordshire District Health
  Authority*
Frank Honigsbaum, *University of
  Birmingham*

Preface

In the face of the relentless rise in health costs, many countries have found the need to set priorities in healthcare. Only in that way can maximum use be made of the limited funds available. However, techniques for prioritizing are uncertain and there is much to be learned by sharing experience. Sweden has taken the initiative in this regard by setting up an official committee to examine priority setting, with instructions to draw on the experience of other countries. This highlights the strong and weak points of various models.

A seminar on priority setting was convened in Stockholm in October 1993, with participants from New Zealand, The Netherlands and the United Kingdom as well as Sweden. Although no one came from the USA, the Oregon model was not neglected. This model has stirred interest throughout the world and some attendees were already familiar with its techniques. The seminar thus included a study of the Oregon model as well as those of the four countries which participated. The section on Oregon was read by Paige Sipes-Metzler, the Executive Director of the Oregon Health Services Commission, who kindly suggested changes and additions.

This report contains the major findings of the seminar. These are supplemented by descriptions of the models existing in each country, in order to provide a perspective for the comparisons that were made. The strong and weak points of each model are then presented, followed by a discussion of the major elements entailed in the priority setting process. Many questions need to be resolved and the report concludes with a presentation of the main ones outstanding.

A list of participants appears on page v. The seminar was organized by Johann Calltorp and Stefan Holmström of the Department of Community Medicine, Huddinge Hospital, Stockholm County Council. The rapporteur was Frank Honigsbaum, a Senior Research Fellow at the Health Services Management Centre, University of Birmingham, which is under the direction of Professor Chris Ham.

The seminar was held over the course of two days, the first at Numberghuset in Stockholm and the second at Huddinge Hospital in the Novum Research Park. Although based on the proceedings, this report has also benefited from a prolonged exchange of views with Dr Stefan Holmström. References to publications and papers relevant to the seminar are listed at the end.

Acknowledgements

The authors and publishers wish to thank the following who have kindly given permission for the use of copyright material.

The Ministry of Welfare, Health and Cultural Affairs in the Netherlands for a diagram for the report of the Dunning Committee on *Choices in Healthcare*.

The Ministry of Health in New Zealand for diagrams from a report of the Core Services Committee on *Core Services 1993/94*.

Reprinted from *Social Science and Medicine*, 37, A Bowling, B Jacobson and L Southgate. (1993) 'Health Services Priorities in Explorations in Consultation of the Public and Health Professionals on Priority Setting in an Inner London Health District' pp. 851–7 with kind permission from Elsevier Science Ltd, The Boulevard, Langford Lane, Kidlington OX5 1BG, UK.

The British Medical Journal for diagrams from a book, *Rationing in Action*, 1993.

Introduction

National models

Oregon

Oregon has led the way in priority setting with the most comprehensive model yet devised. This provides, in priority order, an extensive list of condition-treatment pairs which cover the whole spectrum of medical, mental and dental healthcare. However, large amounts of guesswork went into the process owing to data deficiencies. It is still largely untested as it only started operating in February 1994.

New Zealand

Policy-makers have deviated from the Oregon approach by starting with the premise that existing services are suitable, as they represent the values of past generations of New Zealanders, but that changes might be made in the way resources are allocated and services delivered.

The first step was to take an inventory of existing services, using volume and cost data for the 20 most common conditions to show where changes might be made. This approach pursues the goal of greater efficiency before any restriction is placed on services.

It has been followed by a programme designed to remove uncertainty from waiting times for specialist treatment, using a system of nationally agreed criteria for access to services and for prioritizing patients. In addition, highly specialized services are to be located where they will give the best results: in national and regional centres rather than in local units that may not treat enough patients to maintain competence.

The next step will be to determine when services should be publicly funded. The method proposed is less rigid than the one employed in Oregon and does not exclude any existing services. Rather, using four criteria, an attempt will be made to decide *whether* and *when* a service will be provided.

Effectiveness and cost data will play a part in the process, but much will also depend on assessments of fairness and community values. By using an incremental approach which does not shock the system, New Zealand's policy makers hope to develop a more satisfactory way of shifting resources across healthcare as a whole.

The Netherlands

The Oregon model may be closely followed in the Netherlands if the final package there is not unduly influenced by political considerations. Public provision may be limited to those services which are shown (by means of conclusive outcome studies) to be effective. That could result in the exclusion of over half those currently provided.

Sweden

In Sweden, action has been left to local initiative and a diversity of methods are employed, although the Government has recommended some priority setting principles.

The main aim has been to clear waiting lists and distribute resources more fairly. For the most part, councils have concentrated on resource allocation rather than restriction of services. However, Oregon methods have been used in a few places, such as Gavleborg. There has been virtually no public consultation.

United Kingdom

As in Sweden, local health authorities have been responsible for their own priority setting. Some have adapted Oregon methods and employed novel means of public consultation. The British Government has set targets for reducing the incidence of some high-profile conditions and reducing waiting lists, but has given no guidelines on prioritizing. In particular, it has refused to authorize exclusion of any service, so fund restrictions across the spectrum of care have been prevalent.

General considerations

Priority setting inevitably involves subjective judgements; there is no magic formula to facilitate the process. Oregon tried one based on QALYs (cost per quality adjusted life years) but found cost and outcome data lacking.

Lack of data

At the moment, data is sufficient only to assess priorities within specialties in the form of 'bite-size chunks'. Even then, reliable data exist only for discrete forms of treatment rather than the broader aspects of care. Thus, in the case of heart disease, the cost and outcome of heart operations can be gauged more confidently than efforts concentrated on prevention and rehabilitation.

Values

All five participating countries recognize the need for the development of ethical or public values to influence priority setting. Oregon produced a large number, and similar ones have appeared elsewhere, but there is much uncertainty about how they should be applied to the priority setting process.

Needs assessment

Needs assessment has progressed furthest in the UK, relying mainly on epidemiological studies conducted by medical directors of public health. A common needs project developed in Oxford has been particularly useful since it can be applied directly to the priority setting process. However, implementation has proved difficult and closer provider involvement, particularly by doctors, is considered essential.

QALYs

Oregon was forced to rule out quality of life considerations because they violated federal law which protected the rights of disabled persons. Criticism based on inadequate data and cultural differences has also been expressed in New Zealand, but no similar objections have been registered by official bodies elsewhere. QALYs are likely to be used in the Netherlands, the UK and by some county councils in Sweden.

Age and lifestyle

In all five countries, age and lifestyle have generally been ruled out as considerations determining access to services, but they may be taken into account in assessing outcome. Thus, elderly persons or smokers could be denied heart operations if benefits were judged to be limited. Such decisions are normally left to clinicians.

Clinical guidelines

Guidelines and protocols are used in all five countries as a means of securing more appropriate care. In New Zealand much effort has been devoted to the development of guidelines for 10 core health services (as well as one for disability support services) prepared by consensus conferences involving professionals and lay experts. There are also plans to develop guidelines for primary care.

However, it remains to be seen whether guidelines will be followed, and methods that are acceptable to clinicians need to be devised to monitor the process. In the UK, shared care protocols have been particularly difficult to formulate and even harder to implement because they require the agreement of GPs as well as specialists.

Public consultation

The Swedish have yet to develop a procedure for public consultation, but a variety of methods have been employed elsewhere. Generally, it is recognized that it will take time to persuade the public to accept the need for choices. The most ambitious attempt is planned in the Netherlands where a three-year programme, set forth in considerable detail, will be aimed at influential consumer groups. However, here as elsewhere, it is not certain what action will be taken if the public's views conflict with those of health authorities.

Priority preferences

In all five countries, priority setting has favoured prevention efforts and care for the chronic sick and deprived groups. The idea is to devote more resources to the mentally ill, for example, than to those needing high technology treatment. It remains to be seen whether these priorities will be accepted by the public.

Insufficient outcome data exist to justify the preference shown for the chronic sick and deprived groups. Since outcome data for these services are difficult to obtain, methods based on process may be needed. Thus, a successful outcome for treatment of schizophrenia may be suggested by the extent to which schizophrenics take the drugs required for treatment.

Shift to community care

In Sweden and the UK, a major effort is being made to shift services from hospitals to the community. For this purpose, Sweden needs to increase GP numbers and develop a system of primary care which screens access to specialists. The UK already has a large number of GPs who provide this gatekeeper role and who may only need further training and equipment. However, changes may be required in the concept and organization of general practice in the UK in order to maximize the shift of services.

GP fundholders

In the UK, GPs with a sufficient number of patients can hold budgets of their own. This has created difficulties for health authorities when trying to set priorities. Links between the two are needed to preserve the local provision of core services and ensure the development of co-ordinated plans.

Part 1

Priority Setting
Models: country
comparisons

Oregon

History

Priority setting in Oregon grew out of the funding problems of the public programme Medicaid, which offers healthcare to the poor. Medicaid was created by the federal government, but participation is voluntary and each state administrates its own programme. However, all 50 states now have a programme. Since over half the funds come from Washington, they must follow rules laid down by the federal government. Some forms of care are mandated and cannot be withdrawn.

A poverty level is set by the federal government. Oregon, like many states, found that it could include only 58% of the poor in its Medicaid programme. However, those who were eligible received a wide range of care. In 1987, Oregon decided to extend coverage to 1500 women and children with the aim of reducing the state's high infant mortality rate. To make this possible, the state decided to remove heart, liver, pancreas and bone marrow transplants from Medicaid, because they were an expensive form of treatment. Only cornea and kidney transplants were retained. Cornea transplants were few in number and had low costs and most kidney transplants were covered by a federal programme.

Preparation of a detailed priority list

This led Oregon to try a different approach. The state did not think it fair to single out one expensive procedure and leave others untouched, so it decided to prepare a priority list covering the whole spectrum of care. All the poor would now be covered, but the state legislature would decide how far down the list Oregon could afford to go.

The aim was to define a basic package of care which would apply to everyone, not just the poor. Many people working for small businesses and individuals with high health risks had no health insurance. The first extension would be made to them and then it would be offered to all in employment-covered contracts. Eventually, coverage would apply to 95% of the population under 65, the age at which America's other main public programme, Medicare, takes over. Initially, the list would not apply to the elderly, blind and disabled, but steps have since been taken to include them as well.

A commission of 11 members was created to prepare the list, consisting of five doctors, a public health nurse, a social worker and four consumers of healthcare. All served in a voluntary capacity, but they were aided by a paid staff and other expenses were incurred. The initial cost came to over $500 000, but the total has now risen to nearly $2 million due to revisions.

First methodology

The first attempt to prepare a list relied solely on the use of quality adjusted life years (QALYs). The list covered the whole spectrum of medical, mental and dental healthcare and 1680 procedures were ranked in the form of condition-treatment pairs (eg appendicitis-appendectomy) with the lowest cost QALY at the top and the highest at the bottom. However, this technique produced so many anomalies that the experiment nearly collapsed. Whilst reliable data were available for some discrete procedures, such as heart operations, they were not available for others, particularly the treatment of chronic conditions such as arthritis and schizophrenia. The most serious deficiency was in cost and outcomes.

Development of categories

The Commission then tried an approach which combined a listing by category with condition-treatment pairs ranked within the category that most applied to them.

The categories were ranked in priority order, using 13 values supplied by the public at community meetings held throughout the state. The public was not considered competent to rank the values, so they were listed only according to the frequency with which they were expressed. These were (in order):

1 prevention
2 quality of life
3 cost effectiveness
4 ability to function
5 equity
6 effectiveness of treatment
7 number benefiting (the number of people affected by the condition and benefiting from the treatment)

8 mental health and chemical dependency (considered important enough to rank as an independent value)

9 personal choice

10 community compassion

11 impact on society (most evident with regard to infectious disease)

12 length of life

13 personal responsibility (or the extent to which a person's lifestyle, eg smoking, is responsible for illness).

The Commission then used its own judgement to group these values into three classes:

- essential to basic healthcare
- valuable to society
- valuable to an individual needing the service.

These could be classified as 'essential', 'important' and 'not so important'. Prevention and quality of life appeared under all three headings, whilst number benefiting, impact on society and cost effectiveness were the other three values put in the 'essential' group. Personal responsibility was not included: it was the only value left for future study.

This process resulted in the ranking of the 17 categories of healthcare. Life-saving treatments with full recovery were put at the top, followed by maternity care; treatments with little or no effect were put at the bottom. (See Figure 1 for a useful adaptation of category ranking prepared by Dr Geoffrey Carroll of the UK.)

Disease oriented   Rank   *Health oriented*

Fatal conditions

Treatment prevents death:
  Full recovery 1
                                    2 .. Maternity care
  Residual problems 3
                                    4 .. Preventive care for children
Treatment extends life and quality
  of life 5
                                    6 .. Reproductive services
Comfort care 7
                                    8 .. Preventive dental care
                                    9 .. Adult preventive care (I)

Non-fatal conditions

Acute condition:
  Treatment provides full cure 10
Chronic condition:
  Single treatment improves quality
  of life 11
Acute condition:
  Treatment achieves partial
  recovery 12
Chronic condition:
  Repeated treatments improve
  quality of life 13
Acute, self-limiting condition:
  Treatment speeds recovery 14
                                    15 .. Infertility
                                    16 .. Adult preventive care (II)

Fatal or non-fatal conditions

Treatments provide minimal or no
  improvement in length or quality
  of life 17

Figure 1:   Health Services Commission priorities by category.
(Devised by Oregon Health Services Commission, Portland, USA.)

Insertion of condition-treatment pairs

The next step was to put condition-treatment pairs into their proper categories and list them in priority order. The pairs were first divided into conditions which could be cured and those which could not, followed by a further division into acute and chronic. Since preventive and some other services could not be subjected to cost-benefit analysis, the classification process was confined to 10 categories.

To facilitate the process, the Commission's staff developed a formula based on rates of mortality and quality of well being. Thus, in the first category came fatal acute conditions with treatment resulting in at least a 25% reduction in mortality during the five years following treatment, and with at least 90% of patients returning to a very high quality of life.

Ranking within category was first carried out using a mathematical formula similar to the one used on the preliminary list, but with less weight to cost and more to duration of benefit and quality of well being. This is called 'net benefit' as opposed to the cost benefit approach used earlier.

However, many items were moved out of category to higher or lower rank according to the judgement of the Commission. Intuition and a concern for political realities had to be applied before the list could be completed.

State legislature covers 587 items

By combining similar condition-treatment pairs, the Commission managed to cut the number from 1680 (on the preliminary list) to 709 (as sent to the state legislature). Mental health and chemical dependency conditions had been included in the preliminary list but were not in this one. They were being considered separately and would be added later.

Every citizen regardless of his or her condition, would be entitled to a diagnosis, but funds were available to cover the first 587 items only, which meant that treatment for 122 items at the bottom of the list would not be forthcoming under Medicaid. (See Figure 2 for the ranking of selected items prepared by Frank Honigsbaum of the UK.)

Condition	Treatment	Category	Rank
pneumonia	medical	1	1
appendicitis	appendectomy	1	5
ischaemic heart disease	cardiac by-pass operation	3	149
HIV disease	medical	5	158
imminent death	comfort care	7	164
cancer of uterus	medical and surgical	5	186
end-stage renal disease	medical (dialysis)	5	319
cataract	extraction	11	337
osteoarthritis	hip replacement	11	399
wisdom teeth	surgery	11	480
tonsils and adenoid	surgery	11	494
hernia (no obstruction)	repair	11	504
back pain (spondylosis)	medical and surgical	13	586

All below 587 not funded

Condition	Treatment	Category	Rank
varicose veins	stripping/sclerotherapy	11	616
bronchitis	medical	13	643
cancer (treatment will not result in 10% of patients surviving five years)	medical and surgical	17	688
tubal disfunction	in-vitro fertilization	15	696
haemmorrhoids	haemmorrhoidectomy	17	698
AIDS, end stage HIV	medical	17	702
extremely low birth-weight babies (under 500 gm)	life support	17	708

Figure 2   Ranking of selected condition-treatment pairs. (Devised by Frank Honigsbaum, University of Birmingham, UK.)

Among the excluded items were eight from the 366 in the original 'essential' group, 51 from the 275 in the 'important' group and 68 from the 'not so important' group. On the preliminary list, all the transplants had come near the bottom, but now 12 out of 19 were covered.

Final rankings were greatly influenced by the judgement of the commissioners. Over half the items were moved at least 25 lines from their original position, and about a quarter moved up or down at least 100 lines. This meant that 60 items changed coverage, with 30 moving above line 587 and 30 going below.

The members of the state legislature rejected an attempt to apply the list to their own health insurance plan. However, the main object of the Oregon plan was to extend coverage, not save money. It will cost at least 25% more than current provision and the legislature voted to add sufficient funds despite budget difficulties stemming from restrictions on property taxes.

Federal action forces revision

President Bush was expected to approve the plan, but he rejected it as a result of protests from disabled groups who claimed that it violated the Americans with Disabilities Act 1990. The Commission was told to eliminate any evaluations of quality of life. Dollars saved per life remained an acceptable criterion, but only if it measured the effectiveness of treatment and not the subsequent quality of life. To give an example, a treatment which saved a limb could be placed higher than one which resulted in the loss of the limb, but no consideration could be given to the fact that the patient was left in a wheelchair if the limb were lost.

Two items were specifically challenged: no liver transplant for alcoholic cirrhosis (line 690), and no life support for premature babies with extremely low birthweight (line 708). The former was said to violate the Americans with Disabilities Act since an alcoholic is considered a person with a disability; the latter was considered to be a potential violation of child protection laws.

The revised list

The Commission then produced a new list of 688 items, of which 568 were funded. (That has since changed to 696 items with 565 funded.) All references to quality of life were eliminated, and medical effectiveness (as determined by the treatment's ability to prevent death) was used to rank services, with cost a factor only when treatments were equally effective. Final adjustments were made by the commissioners, who applied 12 subjective criteria ranging from preventive services to public health risk. As with the preceding list, the Commission's judgment was a major factor in determining list priority.

The main changes were as follows: all liver transplants were covered in line 132, the lower ranking (of 690) for alcoholic cirrhosis being eliminated; and treatment for all premature babies under 2500 gm were covered in line 40, eliminating the lower ranking (of 708) for babies under 500 gm.

Clinton approves list

The new Vice-President, Al Gore, strongly opposed the Oregon plan, as did the Children's Defense Fund, the organization with which the new President's wife, Hillary

Clinton, had long been associated. However, President Clinton approved the plan subject to several conditions, the main one being that no more treatments could be cut (above the 568, now 565, line already set by the Oregon legislature) without federal approval.

Principles of the final plan

The Commission realized the aim of those who initiated the plan: it produced a significant shift in priority from curative to preventive services, and from high technology treatments to those concerned with maternity and childcare.

No attempt was made to deal with co-morbidities such as a patient suffering from heart disease as well as diabetes. The extent to which a person should be personally responsible for his or her illness was also excluded. Both were left to further study.

An impressive list of public values were produced, but the community meetings from which they emerged were not representative of the general public. About two-thirds of those who attended were workers employed in the health services, who would be affected by changes in Medicaid.

The plan started operating on 1 February 1994, as a demonstration project. This means that it will be carefully monitored and assessed over a five-year period. During its first month of operation, there was a sharp increase in demand for services under Medicaid. Only 13 000 people were expected to sign up, but in the first two weeks the authorities received 46 000 phone calls and 25 000 applications by mail. This raises the possibility that the plan will cost more than anticipated and more services may have to be withdrawn.

However, the Oregon plan may be overtaken by Clinton's far-reaching health security programme, since that envisages the incorporation of Medicaid within the larger framework. If that proposal is passed, all patients, including the poor, would be entitled to the same package of benefits, including some services not covered in the Oregon plan. Meanwhile, other states have adopted the Oregon procedure in setting priorities under their Medicaid plans.

In any event, the Oregon Health Commission has been saddled with a major new task that could strain its resources. Under an Act passed in 1993, it is now expected to set clinical guidelines for line items. In view of the Commission's shrinking budget, this might only be possible for selected items in the list. It expects to limit preparation to items of clinical significance and, because of the elaborate procedure devised for selection and adoption, to restrict the maximum number to eight every two years. The task will be made more difficult by the departure of one of the most able members of the Commission, Dr Tina Castanares. Her term expired and she has not continued membership.

New Zealand

History

Priority setting in New Zealand operates within the framework of an internal market similar to that of the UK. A split between purchasers and providers was created in July 1993. Purchasers took the form of four appointed regional health authorities (RHAs) with populations raging from 684 000 to 1 079 000, which replaced the 14 elected area health boards that previously combined both functions. RHAs can purchase care from public, private or voluntary providers and since nearly one million of the 3.4 million people in New Zealand have private health insurance, the private sector occupies a more prominent place than in the UK. However, fees and charges apply mainly to primary care (which many pay for directly), so the total amount spent on private insurance is not as great as it would be if more people needed hospital coverage.

Most large public hospitals have become crown health enterprises that operate like companies and make a profit. Smaller communities will have the opportunity to run their local hospitals as community trusts. GPs were encouraged to manage their own budgets, but the profession opposed the move and the Government agreed to continue with open-ended fee for service arrangements for those who opposed controls. Primary care is not free – the government only provides subsidies based on income – and doctors feared that their right to set the upper limits of fees would be restricted if they became budget holders.

Hospital care had traditionally been free in the public sector, but in 1992 charges were introduced for those with high incomes, defined as $NZ28 000 (about £10 000) or over for families and $NZ17 000 or more for single people. The fee was set at $NZ50 per night for 10 nights a year, or a maximum of $NZ500. The public deeply resented the charge, fearing it would lead to privatization, and it was dropped after only 13 months. However, charges still apply to out-patient care for those with high incomes.

Originally, it was proposed to introduce competition into purchasing as well as the provision role. The public was to have the right to choose private health plans instead of the Government one, but this too was dropped. However, public hospitals can now generate income from private patients, a right which did not previously exist. The four RHAs are responsible for purchasing the whole array of care – in the primary as well as the secondary sector – and unlike in the UK, the division of functions extends to the ministerial level, with a new minister having been appointed to oversee public hospitals.

The need to restrict public services

In addition to the introduction of an internal market, the Government finds it necessary to restrict the health services it offers within the public sector. In 1991, health care consumed 7.4% of the gross national product. Although this was not high by international standards – and private spending (18%) accounts for a larger proportion of health expenditure than in the UK – the New Zealand economy has failed to grow over the past 20 years and the rapid advance of medical technology, together with an ageing population, has put increasing strain on public finance. The need for change is not accepted by the opposition Labour party, which vowed to scrap the internal market if it won the general election in November 1993. However, the National Government retained power with a slim majority and the internal market remains.

Although primary care has long been only partly covered by public subsidies, hospital and specialist services are largely free. Certain operations, eg liver transplants, are not performed in New Zealand and a fixed sum has been set aside each year to help people travel overseas for such procedures – currently, to Australia. If this runs out, then many communities make up the shortfall with local fund-raising efforts.

In the past, area boards were expected to provide a comprehensive range of secondary care from the fixed sums they received. As in the UK, each board made its own decisions and priority setting mainly took the form of waiting lists which varied from place to place. For the most part, clinicians decided admission to, and placement on, waiting lists.

The new regional health authorities have inherited this situation. They are also required to purchase secondary care services within fixed budgets. The RHAs are now working co-operatively to develop standardized assessment criteria and a system of priority ranking for access to services in key treatment areas. Whilst access will continue to be restricted to 'those who can obtain the highest net benefit', unfair variation in access around the country is likely to be reduced.

Defining core services

The Government wants to retain the general principle of universal access, but restrict the range of services to an essential core progressively defined according to the benefits services provide. To start the process, the government has indicated that core services will not necessarily be free or immediately available, but that any charges imposed will be affordable and waiting times reasonable.

Recommendations of the Core Services Committee

The Committee took a cautious approach to defining the core. It started from the premise that the services which already existed were necessary and suitable, representing the values and priorities of past generations of New Zealanders, but that changes might be made in the way resources are allocated. The committee noted that the drive to practise defensive medicine is low in New Zealand because 'no-fault' accident coverage applies across the country. New technology had been adopted with caution. There was also said to be no great pressure to prolong life when this was no longer viable.

Since existing services provided the core, the Committee saw its first task as the preparation of an inventory. No detailed analysis has yet been made of disability support services and more data is needed on community care, but from its stock-taking, the Committee found inequities in the provision of primary as well as secondary care and stressed the need for fairer allocation of resources for services like hip replacements and heart operations. In Auckland, 50% of patients paid privately for lens replacement of cataracts, whilst in Northland, the immediately adjoining former area health board, 70% of patients had it done without charge in public hospitals.

By showing not only the unit cost but the volume of treatment for the 20 most common conditions, the Committee was able to demonstrate how savings might be realized for greater efficiency as well as priority setting. For example, the largest cost was due to normal childbirth, with bed stays twice the American average: if only one day were cut, that would be enough to provide a 120 bed hospital (see Figure 3 on page 28).

How should the core be defined? To start the process, a public debate was launched followed by the appointment of an advisory committee to find out how health service money is currently spent and what changes should be made to produce a core service. The committee was asked to make annual recommendations to the Minister of Health, both on how money should be spent and on what terms patients should have access to services. At first, its remit applied only to health services, but it was later extended to cover disability support services as well.

Public reaction

From the public debate came 700 submissions with strong support for the principle of universal access to public services. Criticism was directed at the Government for its failure to consult the public on major decisions already taken. It was repeatedly said that the case for defining the core, as well as the need for an internal market, had not been substantiated, and that not enough information had been provided to

Ranked by: volume

Rank	Volume	Unit cost	DRG cluster	Total cost
1	44 356	2247	Normal birth	99 673 334
2	19 705	1568	Digestive disorders	30 895 725
3	14 269	1594	Asthma and bronchitis	22 743 084
4	11 258	1295	Pregnancy complications	14 579 696
5	7441	2434	Heart and chest pain	18 108 497
6	7234	1175	Abortion with D & C	8 502 348
7	7126	4541	Uncomplicated caesarean section	32 359 025
8	6136	4683	Heart attacks	28 737 375
9	5750	2246	Back problems (without- surgery)	12 913 173
10	5342	10076	Stroke	53 823 354
11	5143	1282	D & C conization	6 595 844
12	5075	3710	Vaginal delivery with complicated diagnosis	18 828 720
13	4992	964	Ear infections and related disorders	4 810 295
14	4870	4690	Chronic obstructive lung disease	22 841 920
15	4788	4963	Heart failure and shock	23 763 039
16	3991	2811	Cataract surgery	11 217 728
17	3785	517	False labour	1 955 904
18	3745	4736	Uterine/adnexa surg non-malig < 70	17 736 940
19	3734	1426	Skin and breast surgery < 70	5 324 410
20	3603	11 517	Knee and hip replacement	41 497 256

Figure 3a: The 20 most common kinds of discharge diagnoses (Devised by the National Advisory Committee on Core Health and Disability Support Services, Wellington, New Zealand.)

enable the public to make sound judgements on how the core should be constructed.

Many people opposed the development of a detailed priority list on Oregon lines, finding it complex, time-consuming, costly and divisive. They wanted to see a more

Ranked by: unit cost

Rank	Volume	Unit cost	DRG cluster	Total cost
1	9	152 644	Extensive burns with surgery	1 373 796
2	6	78 032	Heart transplant	468 194
3	44	48 676	Extensive burns w/o surgery, non-extensive with	2 141 725
4	528	35 500	Extreme immaturity, respiratory distress	18 744 239
5	26	28 839	Mult major joint surgery, lower extremities	749 820
6	466	27 627	Cardiac valve surgery with pump	12 874 054
7	130	22 231	Pancreas, liver and shunt surgery	2 890 080
8	1051	21 428	Heart bypass surgery (CABG)	22 521 177
9	107	20 660	Major head and neck surgery	2 210 658
10	207	20 522	Lymphoma, leukemia with major surgery	4 248 140
11	259	18 483	Amputation for circulatory system except toe	4 786 997
12	37	18 352	Skin graft, debride for endocrinal/metabolic changes	679 029
13	847	15 925	Major reconstructive vascular surgery	13 488 791
14	71	15 503	Kidney transplant	1 100 713
15	221	14 988	Ulcer skin graft or debridement	3 312 410
16	974	14 731	Brain surgery	14 347 673
17	306	14 272	Other cardiothoracic surgery w/o pump	4 367 153
18	642	12 995	Rectal resection	8 342 708
19	1140	12 990	Stomach, oesophagus, duodenal surgery	14 808 451
20	7	12 749	Permanent pacemaker with heart failure	89 243

Notes: Source – PMS database year ending June 1991
Public Hospitals only
Excluding Mental Health Diagnoses

Figure 3b: The 20 kinds of discharge diagnoses that have the highest cost per discharge

Ranked by: Total cost

Rank	Volume	Unit cost	DRG cluster	Total cost
1	44 356	2247	Normal birth	99 673 334
2	5342	10 076	Stroke	53 823 354
3	3603	11 517	Knee and hip replacement	41 497 256
4	7126	4541	Caesarean section w/o complication	32 359 025
5	2597	12 000	Hip and femur surgery w/o joint replacement	31 165 174
6	19 705	1568	Digestive disorders	30 895 725
7	6136	4683	Heart attacks	28 737 375
8	2116	12 050	Major small and large bowel surgery	25 498 598
9	1985	12 261	Premature neonate, except extreme immaturity	24 338 384
10	4788	4963	Heart failure and shock	23 763 039
11	4870	4690	Chronic obstructive lung disease	22 841 920
12	14 269	1594	Asthma and bronchitis	22 743 084
13	1051	21 428	Heart bypass surgery (CABG)	22 521 177
14	5075	3710	Vaginal birth with complications	18 828 720
15	528	35 500	Extreme immaturity, respiratory distress	18 744 239
16	3745	4736	Uterine/adnexa surgery non-malignant <70	17 736 940
17	1868	8057	Degenerative nervous system disorder	15 049 957
18	5750	2246	Back problems w/o surgery	12 913 173
19	466	27 627	Heart valve surgery with pump	12 874 054
20	3030	3420	Lung cancer	10 362 570

Figure 3c: Cost and volume for the 20 most common conditions

general, positive list that would describe in broad categories (such as mental, geriatric and children or perhaps a classification closer to the type used in Oregon) the services that would be provided. However, they wanted enough flexibility to allow regional variation, an important consideration for Maoris, Pacific Islanders and other ethnic groups anxious to have services delivered in a culturally appropriate manner. To the positive list would be added a short negative one, showing specific services to be excluded.

Nevertheless, some people opposed regional variation carried to the lengths that prevail in Britain, where health authorities have responsibility for determining local priorities within the framework of broad national guidance. That was felt to be unjust in a publicly-funded service: people who contribute equally should not be denied access to essential services available elsewhere.

In the process of defining the core, many stressed the need for the development of a broad, ethical framework with widespread public input. Criteria similar to the public values found in Oregon (cost benefit, quality of life, how many people would benefit, prevention) were suggested, and high priority was given to mental health, children's health and integrated community services as opposed to those in the 'hi-tech' sector. In general, the priorities selected called for a shift to prevention and chronic care, but it has proved difficult to secure agreement on which services should be cut.

Waiting lists to be replaced

In its second report, the Committee called for the abolition of waiting lists for non-urgent procedures, replacing them with a booking system under which patients would be given definite dates for specialist services.

Waiting lists presently are too long and vary between regions; they are set up on a 'first come, first served' basis, which the public considers unfair. The booking system is to operate according to nationally agreed criteria so that patients are treated in the same way everywhere. Priority is to be based on the principle of patient need and ability to benefit from the procedure. Such issues as age, cause of disease, earning capacity, ability to cope with pain and number of dependents are not considered key factors. Patients who do not meet the criteria will not be placed on a waiting list, but referred back to their GP for periodic reassessment.

Location of high technology services

The Committee also called for the location of certain high technology services at national or regional level. It deemed this more important than local provision where staff might have an insufficient number of patients to build competence. Kidney transplants would be limited to two units, neonatal care for babies under 1000gm to five units, and liver trans-plants would continue to be provided in Australia but with full public funding now available for nine procedures.

Survey of public opinion

The Committee conducted its own survey of public opinion, drawing on well-attended public meetings with health and disability groups and the responses to a questionnaire from 2500 individuals and community organizations. The priorities suggested were the same as those found in the earlier public debate. However, though the public recognized the need for trade-offs if priorities were to be met, it could not agree on what was to be cut and preferred savings to come from more efficient provision of existing services.

To help the public decide how choices might be made, the Committee has launched another consultation exercise. It starts with the premise that the debate should not be about which services should be publicly funded, but whether and when they should be offered. The key consideration is the benefit of 'a particular service to a particular person at a particular time'.

Four questions need to be answered to determine the core:

- What are the benefits of a service?
- Is it value for money?
- Is it fair?
- Is it consistent with the community's values and priorities?

In answering the first two questions, data regarding outcome and cost effectiveness need to be considered, while the last two involve assessments of equity and morality.

The most important and most complex is the question of fairness. By comparing relative benefits, a way might be found of shifting resources across specialties, but it is proposed that this be done by means of small changes which do not shock the system.

Guidelines for core services

The Committee had not only to start the process of selecting core services, but also to recommend how they should be provided in an effective and fair way. This called for the development of boundary guidelines suggesting what needed to be done in unusual circumstances, but otherwise leaving scope for professional judgement.

Eleven such guidelines were prepared by means of consensus conferences with over 120 professionals and lay experts, covering such services as hip replacements, treatment of end-stage kidney failure and well childcare. The topics chosen had to be ones that were subject to widespread concern, but which were likely to produce a consensus of general application. The age of the patient occupied a prominent place in the treatment of kidney failure, with patients over 75 usually being denied dialysis or transplants, while children under five would not normally be accepted unless there was a prospect of a transplant from a live donor.

During 1993, a further six consensus conferences were held, five concerning disability support services and one, hormone replacement therapy. Advice or guidelines regarding these were included in the Committee's second report and it also called for guidelines to be prepared for primary care. In addition, stress was laid on the need for better co-ordination and integrated planning of health and disability support services.

The Netherlands

History

Priority setting in the Netherlands operates within the framework of an internal market with some characteristics similar to those in place in the UK. However, unlike the British National Health Service, the Dutch system is insurance-based, with 60% of the population covered by mandatory sickness funds and 40% by private funds.

Since 1985, the Dutch Government has been trying to change its health care policy, largely out of concern for the growing costs of care due to an ageing population and the introduction of new technology. The Netherlands is a wealthy country, but health care now consumes 8.6% of the gross national product. Without measures to contain costs, the proportion is expected to rise still further.

The Dekker Committee's insurance scheme

In 1987, a Government committee, the Dekker Committee, proposed compulsory insurance for everyone, but with a basic care package limited to 85% of the health and social services previously provided. More emphasis would be put on prevention and the Government would restrict its role to setting guidelines within which an internal market would operate, leaving insurers to negotiate contracts with providers that would set the parameters and cost of care.

The basic care package would be financed mainly by a percentage premium related to income, but also by a nominal fee per insured person, fixed for each insurer. Since the percentage premium would be deducted from wages, public attention would focus on the nominal fee. Some scope would be left for variation in the range of services provided and this, together with flexibility on costs and method of provision, would enable insurers to offer different packages and premiums. Patients could even insure for special risks to which charges or no-claim discounts might apply. Patients would have a choice of policies, with a change of insurers allowed every two years, and thus insurers as well as providers would be subject to competitive forces.

The Government accepted these proposals but expanded the basic care package to cover 95% of existing services. International treaties limited the extent to which services could be excluded, but how would the basic package be defined?

The Dunning Committee

In 1990, the Dunning Committee was asked to recommend how priorities should be set, with the suggestion that Oregon methods might be employed.

Priority Setting Methods

Dunning did follow Oregon, but only in part. The Committee recommended that four criteria or 'sieves' be used:

- Is the care necessary from the community point of view?
- If so, has it been demonstrated to be effective?
- Is it also efficient, using such methods as QALYs?
- Can it still be left to individual responsibility?

Diagnosis-treatment combinations would be used as in Oregon and they would be listed in priority order within categories based on the nature and severity of the condition and the nature, length and effect of the treatment. However, the final package of necessary care would not be determined by QALYs or assessment of public preferences, but by political considerations.

The community approach

As in Oregon, an *ad hoc* body called the Health Insurance Council could be created to prepare the list. It was recognized that individuals and doctors might take a different view of necessary care, but the Committee felt that the community approach should predominate, defining health as the possibility for every member of society to function normally. This enabled it to urge the protection of services for the chronic sick and other vulnerable sectors such as the elderly, handicapped and mentally ill. As in Oregon, the Dunning Committee felt the need to restrain the use of high technology for the acutely ill. In the interests of equality and community solidarity, it also followed Oregon in ruling out such considerations as the age and lifestyle of a patient as

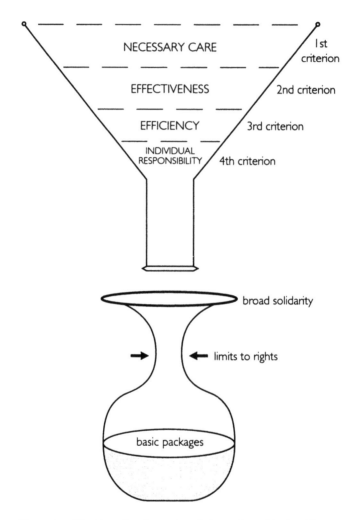

Figure 4: The Dunning Committee's four 'sieves' for health services

grounds for denying treatment. Smokers in the Netherlands would have the same right to heart operations as non-smokers.

Basic care package to be continuously reviewed

The Dutch Cabinet seemed to assume that all care in the basic package needed no further evaluation, but Dunning disagreed. Each service and the conditions under which it was provided would have to be carefully defined, with the possibility of time or expense limits being placed on its application. Essential drug lists should also be prepared, and services which had been included in the basic care package might, upon further investigation, be removed. This would be required where waiting lists proved too long; Dunning thought it inequitable to let them vary too much by locality. If additional funds were not available, then services with lower priorities would be removed from the basic package. As in Britain, waiting lists have hitherto been the normal method by which services were rationed; Dunning proposed the introduction of specific criteria for placement on the lists.

The Committee called for controls over the quality of care, with legal protection for the handicapped and other vulnerable groups likely to lose out under the proposed system of regulated competition. Controls were also recommended over the introduction of new technology, in light of the need to develop wider restraints within the framework of the European Community.

Although supply-side regulation already exists in the Netherlands, with planning of health facilities and a centralized pricing system, Dunning did not find it sufficient. The Committee urged quicker, more effective, action.

Public involvement

It was proposed that the professions would take the lead in defining 'appropriate' care, preparing protocols and guidelines, but that insurers and patient's organizations would also be involved in discussions. However, the Secretary of State for Health wanted a more influential role for insurers and patients in setting norms, which would give the Government final responsibility.

Dunning also had a mandate to involve the public in the process. Opposition to public finance has been growing in the Netherlands and many people believe that only a basic care package should be available to all. Nevertheless, a poll commissioned by the Committee found the majority still opposed to any restriction on treatments, including the most expensive ones. Dunning recognized that it would take time to wean the public to the need for making choices and this instigated a three-year programme aimed at persuading influential consumer groups.

The Government has yet to approve or act on the Committee's recommendations.

Sweden

Healthcare in Sweden is under local authority control: there are 23 county councils and three large municipalities. Since 1992, these have had responsibility for community care, including nursing homes and long-term services for the elderly and disabled.

Compulsory insurance covers everyone, but user fees also have to be paid for all services, except hospital in-patient care, which are partially reimbursed from regionally-organized social insurance funds. Partial reimbursements are also made for the fees charged by private practitioners. In the public sector, the charges for which patients are responsible account for less than 10% of costs. The bulk of the money comes from local authority taxes and payments made into social insurance funds.

Waiting lists have been long in Sweden and productivity low, so in 1992, county councils were required to guarantee care for certain surgical procedures, limiting waits to no more than three months. Failing that, patients will be entitled to go to hospitals in other county councils or in the private sector.

Several county councils have introduced an internal market with a split between purchasers and providers. Falu has GP fundholders who negotiate purchase and sale agreements with the two hospitals located there, but this arrangement is to be phased out.

The Stockholm council reimbursed hospitals on a modified DRG basis to clear waiting lists, but this produced excessive costs and failed to take account of the complexity of patient care. In Sweden, the DRG technique was employed on a flat-rate basis, unlike the varied allowance used in the USA. A switch may be made to specialty-based contracts, but the DRG method has been useful in clearing waiting lists and may be employed again if the need arises.

Steps toward priority setting

Priority setting in Sweden has only just begun and with its healthcare system under local authority control, methods vary greatly. However, a more uniform procedure may develop as the result of action taken by the central Government. Two committees have been appointed, one dealing with the funding and organization of healthcare, the other with priority setting. The latter, which is called the Priorities Commission, is expected to issue a final report by the end of 1994. In October 1993, it published an interim report which set forth a number of principles and proposals for discussion.

Recommendations of the Priorities Commission

As a basis for priority setting, the Commission laid down three principles:

1 Human dignity. This implies that all individuals are of equal value and that none should receive preference in care because of personal characteristics or status in the community. Treatment can be withheld because it might not prove of sufficient benefit, but it cannot be denied solely because of a patient's advanced age, lifestyle or, in the case of premature babies, low birthweight. Similarly, patients who make payments for health services should not be entitled to a higher quality of care, but only to such privileges as a private room while in hospital or other benefits of a 'hotel standard'.

2 Solidarity. Resources should go to those who need them most, particularly to vulnerable groups such as the mentally ill.

3 Efficiency. All other things being equal, the most cost-efficient care should be provided. However, the Commission refused to offer central guidance on an upper limit of expenditure, leaving that to local determination in the event of financial pressures. It recognized that these were a distinct possibility for the smaller budgeting units that would exist in the new system of care started by some county councils, based on an internal market.

The Commission then indicated how priorities might be set at the administrative as well as the clinical level of care. At the administrative level, resources would be allocated on the basis of needs assessment, not the demands of those who shout the loudest, and would apply to treatment groups as a whole rather than to individuals. The latter are subject to decisions made by clinicians who have to adjust the treatment they provide to changing conditions.

The priorities set at both levels are similar and arranged in categories reminiscent of those used in Oregon (and also Norway) but fewer in number – five as opposed to 17.

Priority 1

Everyone should be entitled to a diagnosis, but the highest priority should be given to severe acute diseases which could lead to disability or death. At the administrative level, this category would include treatment for severe chronic disease, palliative terminal care and diseases which entail 'a reduction of autonomy', such as that experienced by the mentally ill. At the clinical level, such treatment would hold a slightly lower priority, life-threatening acute disease receiving preference over everything else.

Priority 2

Prevention measures would come next, including not only those like no smoking efforts targeted at populations as a whole, but also the health screening of individuals. The latter, however, would cover only those which are shown to be cost-efficient. Preventive measures aimed at populations would apply only at the administrative level, since the clinical level is concerned with individuals. However, all forms of prevention might be excluded from the priority classification if, as the Commission suggests, separate financing were provided.

In addition to screening examinations, preventive and rehabilitative services designed for individuals, together with the provision of technical aids, would be included in this priority. This would apply regardless of whether priorities were set at the administrative or clinical level.

Priority 3

This priority includes less severe acute and chronic disease and, like the two which follow, applies at both the administrative and clinical levels. Here, as in all groups, preference would be given to persons likely to receive greater benefit from treatment. However, the Commission warned against giving priority to acute cases which are easily treated as opposed to chronic illnesses where the benefits are less obvious. It offered no guidance as to how this preference might be avoided.

Priority 4

This covers care for reasons other than illness or injury, such as certificates for driving licences, vaccinations for travel abroad, ritual male circumcision and psychotherapy for personality development. It also includes surgery for myopia instead of glasses or contact lenses, assisted fertilization and cosmetic surgery not due to serious injury or deformity (eg the removal of tattoos). In the Commission's view, such measures should be wholly or partly excluded from public provision.

Priority 5

This covers mild disorders where self-care would suffice or where the care provided would serve no useful purpose. The latter would apply particularly to the terminally ill. They would receive palliative care but not treatment of a heroic nature which might only 'prolong the dying process'.

In its terms of reference, the Commission was asked to suggest a basic package of care, but it declined to do so, contending that 'the vast majority of medical care activities should be jointly and equitably funded'.

In this way, the Commission has started to supply the framework through which county councils are expected to set priorities, but this still leaves room for local variation. Until now, the councils have taken the lead in priority setting and they are likely to retain the freedom to try different methods.

General considerations

Oregon list ruled out

Although Swedish interest in priority setting has been inspired by the Oregon example, the county councils involved in the process have thus far seen no need for a detailed list. Oregon had to act because of the growing costs of Medicaid, whereas the Swedish budget system is said to provide strict cost control. However, with health costs at 8.6% of the GNP, this has not been as effective as the budget limits set in the UK.

Family doctor system V. free choice

This situation no doubt points to the need in Sweden for a family doctor system, a major factor behind the relatively low health costs in Britain. At present, primary care is handled mainly by district medical officers working in community health centres, but they cover only about a quarter or a third of demands. Yet, however it is provided, primary care in Sweden can be bypassed by the right of free choice which permits patients to change doctors daily and go to any hospital they choose.

The country is in the process of developing a family doctor system and by 1995 it is hoped to give everyone the chance to enrol with a family doctor and see specialists only on referral. Thereafter, anyone consulting hospitals or specialists directly will have to pay a higher fee. However, a uniform gatekeeper arrangement has been ruled out; the right of free choice, together with a higher regard for specialist as opposed to GP care, is deeply imbedded in Sweden and the politicians feel it must be preserved. (President Clinton has taken the same position in the USA.) If the new arrangement fails to restrain costs, then Swedish Government may have to take a bolder look at priority setting. The country has severe economic problems with an unemployment rate exceeding 9%.

Clearing waiting lists and ensuring fairness

Although priority setting methods vary by locality, the main aim has been to clear waiting lists for critical procedures and distribute resources more fairly. In this respect, it resembles the programme started in New Zealand. Priority setting in Sweden is moving ahead cautiously, with principles and methods proposed for discussion and tried on an experimental basis. Advantage is being taken of experience gained elsewhere and scope allowed for local variation so that different methods may be tested.

The Falu priority list

Work on priority setting at the Falu General Hospital began as early as 1987 and that has made it the centre of attention. However, the techniques employed have aimed only at a fairer distribution of resources across specialties. The goal is to provide a means of classification that could be used by all specialties covering all patients treated, whether as inpatients or out-patients. However, primary care personnel find it geared more to in-patients and that, no doubt, is why it is often described as ' a waiting list model'.

Seven categories of care have been defined in descending order of medical urgency. Acute medical cases needing immediate attention come at the top, and the least urgent at the bottom. The first category covers all forms of emergency care, but excludes patients who are terminally ill, where there is no hope of prolonging their life (or there is only hope of a life of low quality). The bottom category covers those conditions where patients can still live normal or near normal lives. It also includes instances where patients seek 'higher' or more costly levels of care than their conditions warrant.

Out-patients as well as in-patients are classified in these categories, and funds are distributed to specialties in accordance with the proportions found. For patients in neighbouring priority groups, waiting time may be shortened or lengthened depending on the consequences of not giving treatment. Economic factors are also considered. Preventive work is treated separately.

Stockholm study of resource allocation

Work on priority setting has only recently begun in the nine district health authorities of Stockholm, and is concerned solely with finding out how resources are distributed between prevention, acute services and rehabilitation. Initially, the aim is to look at services in 'bite-size chunks' and not to attempt the more difficult task of setting priorities across the whole spectrum of care. Two districts chose cancer and heart disease in a pilot study and this has led to other projects dealing with allergy, mental illness and musculoskeletal diseases.

In pursuing this course, Stockholm has taken a lead from an experiment conducted in the UK, at Southampton, by Chris Ham and Chris Heginbotham, which was published by the King's Fund College under the title *Purchasing Dilemmas*. This approach recognizes that there is no simple method of setting priorities and that priority setting can only be attempted through a process of informed discussion. There is a need to provide as much information as possible about costs, volume, outcome and other relevant data, with regard to all stages of prevention, treatment and rehabilitation.

Gavleborg County Council

Consideration of priority setting began in 1991 and an elaborate model has been prepared, using methods similar to those employed in Oregon. However, it has not yet been implemented as it was proposed only for discussion purposes.

Before priority setting begins, the Council wants to make its delivery system more efficient, particularly by developing primary care services. It also first wants to discontinue treatments with little or no benefit, thereby preparing the way for protocols and guidelines for clinicians to follow. Conditions to be considered would be confined strictly to the health sphere, thereby excluding any form of social work from the priority setting process.

The Council recognizes that priority setting has always existed, but feels the need to make it more explicit through a public process leading to a consensus among politicians, doctors and the public. It has begun by creating an Ethics Committee composed of five doctors representing the major specialties, two nurses and two administrators. These three groups are the main ones involved in fund allocation, with the final decision being taken by the members of the county council.

Ethical principles

In March 1993, the Committee produced a document for discussion, setting forth first the ethical principles to be followed in setting priorities. Four were stressed:

- equality (equal treatment for equal conditions)
- autonomy (the right of patients to refuse treatment)
- the number of patients likely to be affected by the condition
- the need to avoid injury to the patient from treatment.

In addition, the Committee felt it important to think ahead and consider the long-term consequences of medical decisions, not just the immediate effects. It also saw the need to give consideration to the effect of treatment on other persons or patients, as well as the person immediately concerned.

As in Oregon, the Gavleborg Committee ruled out age and lifestyle as a consideration in priority setting. This was presented without qualification, but it is likely that both may be taken into account if they affect outcome. As the discussion progresses, it may be considered that an elderly patient or a smoker could be denied a heart operation if he or she is unlikely to survive or if the treatment will have only a limited effect.

In assessing outcome, the Committee stressed the need for results to be well documented. However, it recognized that this could not always be achieved and that consideration had to be given to another test – a wide consensus as to the positive effects of treatment. In this respect, Gavleborg departs from the Dunning model in the Netherlands, in which the use of 'sieves' means that all care not shown to be effective would apparently be excluded from the basic package.

Services put in four broad categories

In Gavleborg, only a preliminary classification of services has begun, dividing conditions falling in the main specialties into four broad categories depending mainly on the urgency of treatment. Thus, the first group covers treatments that save lives in fatal acute medical cases, and the fourth deals mainly with treatments for relatively minor or self-limiting conditions. The latter is divided into two sections, one covering treatments with documented benefit and the other, those without documented benefit.

For each of these categories, examples of conditions are given, supplied by the doctors involved in each specialty. Thus far, only a few have been indicated, but the list will be expanded in a more formal way when the medical specialists are given the opportunity to discuss and challenge each other in an attempt to secure consensus. After that, they will have to convince the politicians that the list is right, as the final decision will be made by the members of the Gavleborg council.

This method resembles the one used in Oregon but with fewer categories (four instead of 17) and with the classification of conditions being determined by doctors from the various specialties rather than by an independent body using a more formal technique, including the application of an algorithm and the consideration of net benefit data. In addition, and more importantly, Gavleborg gives politicians the final say over list priority, whereas Oregon confined their authority to funding (ie deciding how far down the list the state could afford to go).

As in Oregon, the classification of preventive measures proved troublesome. In Oregon, they were divided into two broad age groups – children and adults – whereas in Gavleborg, they are classified according to the seriousness of the condition with which they are associated. Thus, preventive measures against serious contagious conditions fall in the first category; maternity and paediatric health checks, along with cervical screening, fall in the second; and general health checks fall in the fourth.

The Vasterbotten model

Priority setting here was led by a councillor who, in 1984, became the subject of media attention when she questioned the wisdom of giving treatment to extremely low birth-weight babies. Most paediatricians did not support her, but she did not lose her seat on the council and she persuaded her colleagues to start a new process which is to be implemented (not just proposed for study or discussion). In this respect, Vasterbotten appears to have gone further than other councils in deciding when choices must be made.

The procedure consists of two parts:

1 The doctors and other health personnel provide rele-vant information regarding treatment.

2   The politicians use their own ethical scale of priorities to decide whether it should be given.

The information required covers:

- the number of people affected by the health problem
- whether there is an alternative to the measures suggested for dealing with it
- the likely effects of treatment
- the necessity for treatment
- the question of equity (whether it would be fair to withhold it on social or geographical grounds)
- costs
- a recommendation for a practical course of action.

The politicians then apply an ethical scale (see Figure 5) with greatest weight attached to the seriousness of the condition and then, in descending order, treatments that involve groups that are weak and cannot speak for themselves (eg the mentally ill), cost-effective treatments, treatments whose effects are well documented and, lastly, to treatments that can easily be carried out.

The age and lifestyle of the patient will not be considered in the rationing process, nor will the fact that the treatment involved is new. Patients over 65 will not be denied hip replacements, but other treatments (such as expensive heart operations) may be withheld if few benefits are expected.

This procedure is designed to deal with particular treatments, but the council also wants it to be used to cover the whole process of resource allocation, including the preparation of budgets and an assessment of results.

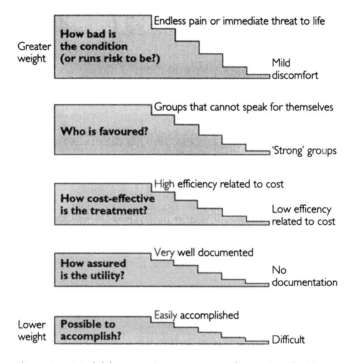

Figure 5: Model for assessing treatment values using the Vaster-botten ethical scale

The need for public consultation

Priority setting in Sweden has thus far failed to make provision for public consultation. Politicians have been fearful of raising the issue because of its electoral consequences. Gavleborg Council sees the need for a public process, but it is unclear how far this has progressed.

All that has been attempted thus far were six radio programmes and a pilot study of 1500 people who were asked to respond to a questionnaire sent through the post. The initiative for this work has come from Dr Stefan

Holmström of the Department of Community Medicine in Stockholm. He has also supplied budget information to patients in the south-east district as part of an effort to solicit the values the public wants to apply to priority setting.

Holmström is surprised at the extent to which the public is both informed and ready to approach the subject, but feels the need to proceed cautiously. He has started training sessions for politicians so that they know how to deal with the media.

United Kingdom

Priority setting in the UK operates within the framework of a comprehensive National Health Service (NHS) open to everyone. It is financed mainly by taxation, so no insurance or means tests apply. Some user charges are imposed, principally for prescriptions and dental treatment, but not for medical or hospital care.

All forms of health services are provided, yet the NHS consumes only 6% of the gross national product, one of the lowest rates in the developed world. This is due not only to central government control, which enables limits to be imposed on total spending, but to a gatekeeper system under which GPs determine access to specialists. Everyone is entitled to GP care, but for the most part, hospital and specialist services are dependent on GP referrals and the resources available for secondary care.

These resources have never been sufficient to meet demand. Waiting lists for hospital care have existed since the NHS's inception in 1948 and age or other restrictions have been imposed on expensive forms of treatment such as renal dialysis. All such restrictions are set locally, dependent on the resources available and the decisions made by individual health authorities. National targets have been set for reductions in some conditions, but no rules or guidelines have been imposed.

A national target was set for waiting lists with all health authorities expected to clear those waiting more than two years. The aim was largely realized but resulted in longer waits for some patients with serious conditions and a programme is now being devised to ensure quicker attention for them.

Creation of an internal market

Until 1991, local decisions were in the hands of health authorities that had provider as well as resource allocation duties. They not only determined how funds would be spent, but administered the hospital and community services which financed them. So many problems were associated with provider duties that purchasing decisions never received the attention they deserved.

Generally, funds were allocated on an historical basis, with most of the money going into the acute sector. Despite national exhortations, it proved difficult to shift resources to the four 'priority' groups – the elderly, mentally ill, mentally handicapped and physically disabled. Similarly, a programme designed to shift resources from over-provided to under-provided areas had limited success.

In 1991, the NHS was reorganized so that purchasing duties were separated from providing duties and an internal market created. Now, nearly all hospital and community services are in the hands of self-governing trusts, while health authorities confine their attention to deciding how resources will be allocated. This has enabled the purchasing function to receive the attention it deserves and paves the way for significant shifts to be made in the way money is spent.

Primary care has traditionally been in the hands of separate authorities, but it is now the responsibility of commissioning agencies that cover the whole spectrum of healthcare. Soon the authorities themselves will be combined and that will facilitate a shift of resources, where needed, to prevention and primary care.

One link remains unsolved. GPs with a sufficient number of patients (originally 11 000 but now 7 000) can hold budgets of their own. With their medical expertise they are thought to be more attuned to patient demands and can drive a harder bargain with trusts than with health authorities.

However, they cannot assess needs as effectively or take account of the services required for a whole community. As fundholding spreads, fewer funds will be under the control of health authorities and they will find their room for manoeuvre increasingly restricted. Core services provided by local providers could be threatened if fundholders referred patients elsewhere.

If the purchasing function is to develop satisfactorily, then either links will have to be formed with fundholders or their place must be taken by the development, already underway in some areas, of purchasing commissions embracing all GPs. This is welcomed by non-fundholders who have been aroused by the development of a two-tiered system which enables fundholders to jump waiting lists and secure benefits denied to the patients of other GPs.

Managing the internal market

Under the internal market, trusts compete for health authority contracts and those that fail to win them may not survive. However, some restraints are applied at regional level so as to ensure the continuance of local provision. The internal market is thus not left to the free play of competitive forces, but is managed.

For the past two years, this has held purchasers to a 'steady state' so that high cost hospitals have not been imperiled by the loss of contracts. Now, however, purchasers are being pressed to demand cheaper or better services and shift resources to prevention, community services and primary care. These are all sectors where the need is great, where more appropriate delivery of services could be provided and where gains in efficiency may be realized.

To promote the process, a freer rein is to be given to market forces. The 14 regional health authorities have hitherto acted as the restraining force; now, they are to be phased out, their functions being combined with the eight regional offices charged with the overseeing of trusts. This will place purchasing as well as providing activities under the wing of a single agency, but with smaller staffs planned at regional level, that may give too much freedom to competitive forces and weaken the concept of a 'managed' market. At the district level, the purchaser-provider split remains and purchasing authorities may be tempted to abandon the local provision of core services in the quest for lower costs.

Funding problems

Purchasing authorities have found their room for manoeuvre restricted by funding shortages. Fewer than one in three have money available for growth purposes this year and that means resources can only be shifted by cutting services or operating them more efficiently.

As a result, the 'priority groups' have not realized the gains they were intended to receive from purchasing plans. However, it has been possible to shift some resources to primary and community care. In addition, the operation of the internal market is starting to correct geographical inequities. London, which has long been held to be over-provided, is certain to experience the hospital closures that earlier attempts failed to secure.

Priority setting by health authorities

Thus far, priority setting has left considerable room for discretion, but only at district level. The Department of Health sets targets for district health authorities to aim for, but has not ruled out the provision of specific services. Regional health authorities have been similarly constrained; when one attempt to have patients awaiting certain treatments (repair of varicose veins, removal of tattoos, excision of lumps and bumps, extraction of wisdom teeth and in-vitro fertilization) removed form the lists, the Department of Health rescinded the decision. The Act which created the NHS calls for a comprehensive service and that statute, ministers maintain, must be upheld.

Nevertheless, district health authorities have been free to exclude services if they wish, and some have chosen to drop treatments like tattoo removal and in-vitro fertilization. Clinicians also exercise considerable discretion; some surgeons have refused to perform heart operations on smokers if they thought the treatment would not be beneficial. Similarly, elderly patients may be denied renal dialysis or other expensive treatment if poor outcomes are anticipated. Here, the assessment of outcome is said to be critical; treatment, the Department of Health maintains, is not denied because of age or lifestyle alone.

Before the internal market was created, health authorities tended to set priorities in accordance with pressures emanating from two directions: from above came funding and health targets set by the Department of Health and regional health authorities; from below came the demands of clinicians seeking sufficient resources for their specialties. Under the internal market system, health authorities are expected to take a wider view of purchasing and to look in other directions. They have been urged to seek the public's views and also to take account of the economic benefits, or cost-effectiveness, of treatments (see Figure 8 on page 85).

Study of six leading health authorities

To what extent have these aims been realized? How did health authorities go about setting priorities after the internal market was created? To answer these questions, a study, supported by the Department of Health, of six leading health authorities was conducted under the direction of Professor Chris Ham of the University of Birmingham. The six authorities selected were held to be those which were likely to have made the most progress in setting priorities. It was found that each has its own approach and that a variety of methods were employed.

By and large, few changes had been made. Restrained by calls to keep a 'steady state', health authorities did not find it timely to make more than a modest shift in resources. To the extent that reallocations were realized, they tended to favour prevention and community services. This was particularly the case with those authorities faced with the contraction or closure of hospital services. They found it important to sponsor proposals that promised to support and extend the range of primary care.

However, this proved difficult in areas with uneven standards of general practice. GPs under the NHS operate as independent contractors, paid largely on a capitation basis but with extra fees for special services (such as minor surgery or immunizations) and reimbursements for practice expenses. Many need retraining before they can assume a wider range of care duties and, in London particularly, improvements are needed in practice premises.

Needs assessment: Oxfordshire

The priority setting procedure typically begins with an assessment of needs, led by directors of public health. A particularly practical approach was the common needs project adopted in Oxfordshire. Six priority areas (coronary heart disease, anxiety and depression, accidents, cancer, disablement, elective surgery) were chosen for study on the basis of the following criteria:

- frequency or severity of the problem
- spectrum of services covered
- range of service options and potential for changing the way treatment is provided
- cost and frequency of use of services
- services involving different providers.

Initially, no change was made in the level of resources devoted to each priority; instead, consideration was given to the way funds were distributed within the variety of services offered. Thus, in the case of one of the priorities chosen – heart disease – it was possible to spend less on in-patient care and more on rehabilitation.

An attempt was made to determine the most effective and economic way of delivering services. The following issues were tackled:

- day care versus in-patient care
- limits on expensive treatment for severe cases
- health or social service responsibility for long-term disability
- provision of services by nurses or other ancillary personnel in place of doctors
- more money devoted to prevention instead of treatment
- early rather than late intervention to forestall the onset of serious illness
- abandonment of ineffective procedures
- more equitable provision of services across the county and to particular client groups.

Implementation of this programme proved difficult. It was impeded by a severe deficiency of relevant information and provider resistance. Hospital consultants participated in the groups that prepared the plans, but were reluctant to change the way they worked.

The same problem arose in the implementation of service agreements. In place of the block contracts prevalent elsewhere, the authority negotiated separate service agreements with 70 providers which tended to focus attention on detailed clinical issues. This should benefit purchasers because service targets and costs can be set more precisely, but for implementation to succeed, the co-operation of provider management is essential. That is a goal which the authority has set for the future.

The value of the Oxford approach is that it links needs assessment closely with resource allocation instead of leaving managers to decide how a broad epidemiological framework can be used to determine purchasing decisions. At the moment, the method is restricted to 'bite-size chunks' within specialties, but as the process becomes more sophisticated, it may be possible to develop techniques for shifting resources across the whole spectrum of care.

Cost-effectiveness

In setting priorities, little use has been made of data dealing with cost-effectiveness. Only a few studies of particular conditions are available and some are not all that relevant to purchaser needs. More studies are to be prepared with the support of the Department of Health. The need is not only to provide data but to supply it in a form that can be easily digested by purchasers.

With this data, it may be possible to secure the more efficient use of resources and thus avoid, or at least delay, the need to exclude specific services. However, to carry out such a programme requires the consideration of various levels of clinical priority. Figure 6 illustrates the Essex approach to this problem as devised by Dr Geoffrey Carroll. In the UK, much interest has focused on level 2, shifting care from hospitals to the community, and on level 5, the development of protocols and guidelines.

In setting guidelines and protocols, the predominating principle is the appropriateness of a treatment. That is considered more important than the effectiveness or efficiency of the service provided. However, protocols have proved difficult to formulate and even harder to implement.

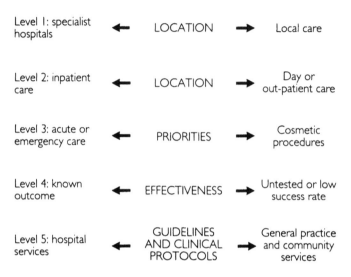

Level 1: specialist hospitals	←	LOCATION	→	Local care
Level 2: inpatient care	←	LOCATION	→	Day or out-patient care
Level 3: acute or emergency care	←	PRIORITIES	→	Cosmetic procedures
Level 4: known outcome	←	EFFECTIVENESS	→	Untested or low success rate
Level 5: hospital services	←	GUIDELINES AND CLINICAL PROTOCOLS	→	General practice and community services

Figure 6: A method of determining clinical priorities, devised by Dr Geoffrey Carroll for North-Essex District Health Authority

This applies particularly to shared care protocols (such as with diabetes and asthma) since they require acceptance by GPs as well as consultants.

Public consultation

Much effort has gone into finding means of involving the public. One authority in London carried out a ranking exercise of 16 treatments and found the public's view in some cases differing significantly from that of doctors. Figure 7 on page 68 shows the results of this exercise.

This raises the question of whose views should prevail. That issue is undecided and is likely to be the subject of considerable debate. From surveys that have been made, it would appear that the public wants the medical profession to take primary responsibility, but politicians think priority setting is considered too important to be left to doctors. If hard choices are to be accepted, then public involvement is required.

Based on the Oregon experience, public consultation may be of greatest use in setting the values that determine priorities. If the public is asked to rank treatments, then relevant information is needed so that informed choices can be made. Thus, a much lower priority might be assigned to neonatal care for babies of extremely low birthweight if the limited benefits of treatment were made known.

The Public Health Forum and use of key informants in Mid-Essex

Led by Dr Geoffrey Carroll, a Director of Public Health, inspired by the Oregon example, the Mid-Essex (now North Essex) District Health Authority has used a variety of techniques to consult the public. Two are noteworthy: a Public Health Forum was created to debate priorities on a regular basis, and a rapid appraisal technique was used to obtain from key informants the views of people not normally concerned with health issues. The Forum was composed not only of groups representing patients but of provider staff and health authority representatives. For the rapid appraisal exercise, 30 key informants were interviewed, all of whom were well placed by their work or social role to gauge the views of the wider public. They included professionals (GPs, social workers, teachers and police) and leaders of voluntary organizations (play groups, youth work and clubs for elderly people) as well as informed individuals (postmen, hairdressers, chemists and other local shopkeepers).

An attempt was made not only to gauge the values the community held about healthcare, but also to determine the

Mean priority ranks (in order of priority 1–16, 1 = highest, 16 = lowest)

Services/treatments	Public	GPs	Consultants	Public health doctors
Treatments for children with life-threatening illness (eg leukaemia)	1	5	2	9
Special care and pain relief for people who are dying (eg hospice care)	2	4	4	8
Medical research for new treatments	3	11	8	11
High technology surgery and procedures which treat life-threatening conditions (eg heart/liver transplants)	4	12	12	12
Preventive services (eg screening, immunization)	5	6	7	4
Surgery to help people with disabilities to carry out everyday tasks (eg hip replacements)	6	8	5	5 equal
Therapy to help people with disabilities carry out everyday tasks (eg speech therapy, physiotherapy, occupational therapy)	7	7	10	5 equal
Services for people with mental illness (eg psychiatric wards, community psychiatric nurses)	8	2	1	1 equal

Figure 7: Results of a public priorities survey in the City and Hackney, 1992. Source: Bowling J, Jacobson B and Southgate L. (1993) Health service priorities: Explorations in consultation of the public and health professionals on priority setting in an inner London health district. *Social Science and Medicine*, **37**: 851–7

Mean priority ranks (in order of priority 1–16, 1 = highest, 16 = lowest)

Services/treatments	Public	GPs	Consultants	Public health doctors
Intensive care for premature babies who weigh less than 1 1/2 lb and are unlikely to survive	9	13	13	15 equal
Long stay care (eg hospital/nursing home for the elderly)	10	3	6	10
Community services/care at home (eg district nurses)	11	1	3	1 equal
Health education services (eg campaigns encouraging people to lead healthy lifestyles)	12	10	11	5 equal
Family planning services (eg contraception)	13	9	9	1 equal
Treatments for infertility (eg test tube babies)	14	14	14	15 equal
Complementary/alternative medicine (eg acupuncture, homeopathy, herbalism)	15	15	16	13 equal
Cosmetic surgery (eg tattoo removal, removal of disfiguring lumps and bumps)	16	16	15	13 equal
Number of respondents	322–335	63–66	112–116	4–6*

*Little can be construed from this sample as the numbers were very small

Figure 7: continued

priorities it assigned to different forms of care. This exercise and others were carried out with the co-operation of the Community Health Council (a statutory body which represents patient interest in the district). Elsewhere, some councils have been reluctant to participate, and are fearful of being involved in the priority setting process.

Growth money and health gain

The widest scope for priority setting exists with growth money, funds which are available for realizing what is called 'health gain'. Here there are no vested interests to consider and proposals can be restricted to areas deemed worthy of development. A variety of methods are used to prioritize proposals, and with increasing sophistication they may one day provide techniques for shifting resources across healthcare as a whole.

City and Hackney: two-stage priority scoring

One authority (formerly City and Hackney, now East London and City) used a two-stage scoring method to assess the proposals it received. In the first stage, bids were ranked on the basis of needs assessment, with greatest weight being attached to services which responded to local needs. Then a short list was prepared and proposals were ranked as follows:

- robustness or the extent to which the   0–3
  proposal can be implemented
- promotion of equity   0–1
- evidence of effectiveness or cost   0–2
  effectiveness

- collaboration with or integration   0–3
  with primary care
- prioritized by the Community   0–1
  Health Council
- prioritized by local GPs   0–1
- other possible or more   0–5
  appropriate sources of funding   (negative score)

Thus, the greatest weight was attached to other funding methods, using a negative score as high as five to cancel out the other weightings. The scores were first determined by the Director of Public Health and then discussed by the purchasing team and the members of the health authority.

Wandsworth

Another authority (Wandsworth) employed a single stage procedure with five criteria weighted as follows:

- potential for health gain   40
- improves quality of service   20
- in accordance with local views   20
- achievability in current year   15
- in accordance with national and regional priorities   5
                                                                  ───
                                                                  100

Here potential for health gain covered a variety of benefits including length of life as well as quality. Ranking was carried out by the non-executive members of the health authority as well as the staff on the purchasing team. They also agreed on a list of priorities to be prepared.

Empirical development

Priority setting in the UK is thus proceeding in an empirical manner, with decisions and methods left to local determination. Health authority managers would welcome greater involvement from national politicians, but it is widely recognized that priority setting cannot be a scientific process.

At present, data are available only to inform discussion on the allocation of resources within specialties in the form of 'bite-size chunks'. Even then, the information is confined mainly to discrete forms of treatment, such as heart operations, rather than the broader aspects of care, such as prevention or rehabilitation. That makes the allocation of resources across the whole spectrum of care a much more difficult process and reforms are therefore proceeding in a cautious and incremental manner.

Although much interest has been shown in the Oregon experiment and some techniques borrowed from it, no attempt has been made to compile a detailed list. In some places, specific services have been withdrawn, but the more common procedure is to reduce funds, leaving some treatment in place across the whole spectrum of care. To the extent that any general direction exists, priorities favour shifts to prevention and community care, but thus far little has been achieved in that department.

To help health authorities set priorities at a local level, the Department of Health has supported a series of projects through its research and development programme. This includes the establishment of a clearing house on healthcare outcomes, publication or reports summarizing evidence on the effectiveness of different interventions, and preparation of epidemiologically based reviews of health needs. These and other initiatives are intended to promote knowledge based purchasing within the NHS and to ensure that resources are targeted in a way which achieves the greatest health gain for the population. Of particular importance is the Cochrane Centre at Oxford which is developing a database on clinical effectiveness. This works in association with the NHS Reviews and Dissemination Centre at York which is responsible for establishing a database on cost effectiveness. The research and develpment programme has also identified health technology assessment as a priority and has provided funds to enable new and existing technologies to be evaluated.

Part 2

Ideas, Methods
and Problems
in Priority Setting

Comparative Evaluation of the National Models

Oregon

Oregon has attempted the most ambitious programme, producing a list which covers the whole spectrum of care. This provides a means of shifting resources across specialties, a technique not yet duplicated elsewhere. It is also the furthest advanced, with operation starting this year. Much may be learned from the experience if offers.

However, owing to data deficiencies, a good deal of guess-work went into its production and some feel that a list of this magnitude (over 600 items) provides too rigid and too mechanical an approach to priority setting. It may also prove difficult to operate since, extensive as the list is, it does not cover the full range of possible diagnoses. Clinicians may find it hard to locate the appropriate line items for the conditions they treat. Moreover, for the system to operate satisfactorily, protocols or guidelines are needed for each item on the list, and that task may prove too ambitious to complete.

In other countries (discussed below), efforts are at an earlier stage, with attempts still being made to devise a satisfactory method of priority setting.

New Zealand

New Zealand provides the sharpest contrast with Oregon. It started with an inventory of services, and aims, initially at least, only to produce a shift in the way resources are allocated. This approach makes possible the pursuit of greater efficiency before any attempt is made to restrict services, a procedure which Oregon did not follow.

However, in New Zealand a core service remains to be defined. Although the public recognizes the need for this, it has yet to accept a cut in services. Thus, service restrictions as such have been ruled out; rather, the aim will be to decide whether and when to provide 'a particular service to a particular person at a particular time'. This could provide more flexibility in service provision than the priority list prepared in Oregon.

It is also hoped to devise a more satisfactory method of shifting resources across healthcare as a whole, relying not only on subjective assessments of fairness and community values, but also on clinicians' judgements about the service impacts and health gains achievable by progressively increasing or decreasing funding in service areas.

The Netherlands

In the Netherlands, Oregon methods have been followed only in part. The Dunning Committee recommended that a priority list be prepared, but it specifically gave precedence to political considerations which have played a lesser role in the Oregon process. The four 'sieves' clarify the issues for the public and the final one – which excludes services that can be left to individual responsibility – adds a novel criterion to those employed in Oregon, which should prove generally acceptable.

However, the Committee has apparently taken a stricter view of 'effective' care than may be politically feasible. To pass through this sieve, the care provided must be of *proven* effectiveness, a test which fewer than half of all health services can pass. This could obstruct the committee's desire to protect the chronic sick and vulnerable groups such as the mentally ill, since many of the services provided to such patients have yet to prove their worth.

One of the strongest aspects of the Netherlands model is the importance it attaches to public consultation. The detailed three-year programme it has devised has been spelled out in considerable detail and may eventually wean the public to the need for hard choices.

Sweden

With healthcare under local authority control, the Swedish system allows room for flexibility and experimentation in the priority setting process. Everywhere it is still at an early stage of development, which provides the opportunity for a variety of methods to be demonstrated and tested. Two are notable.

By pursuing the 'bite-side chunk' approach pioneered in Southampton, England, Stockholm Council confines its efforts to conditions for which adequate information can be obtained to make informed decision. It recognizes that priority setting inevitably involves subjective judgement; there is no magic formula to facilitate the process. It believes that only by a step-by-step approach can methods be devised that will enable resources to be allocated across the whole spectrum of care.

Gavleborg Council follows a broader approach, more in line with the Oregon model. It aims to construct a priority list covering the main specialties, but is proceeding in a cautious manner, giving the doctors involved a chance to reach agreement on the priorities assigned. In addition, in contrast to the Netherlands, it recognizes the difficulty of proving effectiveness and will accept the existence of a wide consensus as to the worth of treatment.

Swedish authorities have yet to offer scope for public consultation as politicians fear the consequences. None of the county councils have devised a programme. This is the country's greatest failing in the priority setting process.

Now that the first report of the Swedish Priorities Commission has been issued, guidance has been offered to local authorities which may quicken the pace of priority setting. Aided by expert advisers and drawing on extensive documentation, the Commission presented a report which, though intended for discussion, may be widely implemented. It stresses the need for effective as well as efficient care, while rejecting age, lifestyle or low birthweight as general grounds for prioritization. Such factors may be considered only if they affect the outcome of care in an individual case.

By distinguishing between priorities at administrative and clinical levels, the Commission recognizes the different considerations involved. It is particularly anxious to secure adequate provision for vulnerable and disadvantaged groups, such as the chronic sick, the mentally ill and those in terminal care. To ensure that this happens, it stresses the need for adequate provision to be made at administrative rather than clinical level, listing in descending order five groups. The highest priority is being given to those who are severely or terminally ill with life-threatening acute disease or disabling chronic disease. Preventive and rehabilitative services come next, followed by the treatment of those with less severe acute or chronic disease. In the fourth group is care for reasons other than disease, such as assisted fertilization or cosmetic plastic surgery. Finally, the lowest priority is given to minor ailments which patients can handle themselves.

United Kingdom

In the absence of national direction, the UK's system also leaves room for local flexibility and a number of interesting methods have emerged. However, whereas a central Government committee in Sweden has recommended priority setting principles for local authorities to follow, the British Government refuses to do more than set targets for reduction in health conditions and waiting lists. Furthermore, though it has refused to exclude services itself, it has left district health authorities free to do so, thereby producing regional disparities which undermine long-standing efforts to achieve uniform provision.

The process of needs assessment has progressed furthest in the UK, in most places in the form of a broad epidemiological framework, but Oxford's common needs project provides a means of linking this more closely with purchasing decisions. Budgets, however, are also held by an increasing number of GPs and this threatens to restrict the ability of health authorities to make sound purchasing decisions or maintain core services. Only New Zealand, of the other four countries, has offered the same arrangement, but few doctors, if any, have adopted it so far.

A variety of methods have been used to set priorities for growth money – ie funds available for service developments – and these may lead to better techniques for shifting resources across the spectrum of healthcare. In general, funding has tended to favour prevention and community care, but some means of assessing outcome is needed if the preference is to be maintained.

Novel methods of consulting the public have been devised, though a ranking exercise for 16 treatments showed the need for relevant information if informed choices are to be made.

Key Elements of Priority Setting

Ethical principles

Before priority setting can begin, it is generally recognized that there is a need to establish ethical principles to underline the process. In Oregon, these were developed from public values expressed at community meetings and were used to rank the categories in which condition-treatment pairs were listed. However, the extent to which the values affected priority ranking was determined by an expert body rather than the public and thus could be said to have been carried out in a somewhat arbitrary manner. Oregon nevertheless succeeded in relating such values to the priority setting process, a link which has not been clearly established elsewhere.

Inventory of services

To start the process, New Zealand policy-makers took the view that they should look first at the country's existing array of services, listing the most common ones according to cost. This approach assumes that the principle aim is to make provision more efficient before any attempt is made to restrict services. It may reveal, as indicated by data from New Zealand, that more money can be saved by reducing bed stays for high volume, low cost treatments than by cutting the number of expensive procedures.

Needs assessment

Before priorities can be assigned, means must be found of determining the need for healthcare. Health authorities in the UK do this by carrying out broad epidemiological studies, but more detail may be desirable to identify pockets of deprivation. Means must also be found of linking needs more closely with purchasing decisions – the methods devised at Oxford show how it can be done.

Competitive pressures

Priority setting is subject to a number of conflicting pressures, as set forth in the model taken from the UK in Figure 8. In the past, most pressures have come from above (national or regional sources) and from below (doctors and others who provide services). As the process becomes more explicit, pressure will also come from the public on the one hand and an increasing array of economic data on the other. Priority setting involves the difficult task of reconciling these conflicting pressures.

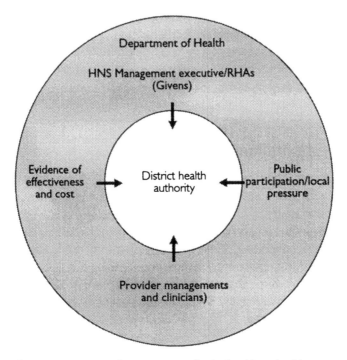

Figure 8: Sources of pressures on district health authorities (Devised by Chris Ham and Chris Heginbotham.)

Public consultation

A number of ways of consulting the public have been tried in the UK and a detailed consultation programme, to be carried out over a three-year period, has been prepared in the Netherlands. There is little to be learned from Oregon since its community meetings failed to attract a representative cross/section of the public.

Much more work needs to be done to devise satisfactory methods, but one point is clear: the public should not be asked to rank treatments unless supporting data are provided. Only then can informed choices be made. Although the public may take a different view of priorities than doctors or managers, it is generally felt that its views cannot be ignored since public acceptance will be needed if hard choices have to be made.

Economic data

Economic data are used to determine the effects of treatments and whether they are worth their cost. Although efforts are being made to increase information, data are still lacking for many procedures, particularly those dealing with chronic conditions. The Dutch are apparently taking a strict view of the effectiveness of treatment, ruling out all procedures for which no positive data are available, but Gavleborg council in Sweden is willing to accept evidence where a wide consensus exists.

Age and lifestyle have been generally ruled out as considerations determining priority, but clinicians may take them into account when assessing outcome. More controversial is the treatment of quality adjusted life years (QALYs). These have been declared violations of federal law in the USA, but they are increasingly used elsewhere.

Range of care covered

Oregon is unique in that it attempted to set priorities for all healthcare under its Medicaid plan for the poor. Elsewhere a more modest approach is being followed. In Stockholm it was decided to limit the process to 'bite-size chunks' within specialties, determining the extent to which resources could be shifted between prevention, treatment and rehabilitation.

However, as was found in Oregon, it is widely recognized everywhere that there is no magic formula by which priorities can be set. No matter which method is used, a good deal of guesswork and judgement must go into the process. As has been realized in New Zealand this may rule out the feasibility of sudden or sweeping change, suggesting instead the desirability of gradual movements in resource allocation.

Priority preferences

In setting priorities, a strong preference has been shown everywhere for more resources to be devoted to prevention and community care, as well as to the chronic sick and vulnerable groups such as the mentally ill. Too much, it is felt, goes into high technology services for the acutely ill.

However, outcome data justifying this preference are lacking and in some places the public has taken a different view. With the Oregon plan starting this year, it may soon be possible to assess the extent to which this priority will be accepted.

Shift from hospital to community care

Efforts are being made everywhere to shift care from hospitals to less costly community services. To facilitate this, the Swedish want to expand their GP corps. However, their existing system, which allows direct access to hospitals and specialists, precludes the development of a gatekeeper role which in the UK does so much to reduce health costs. Despite universal coverage and comprehensive provision, costs in the UK as a proportion of gross national product are among the lowest in the developed world.

However, if the full potential of community care is to be realized, then changes may be needed in the concept and organization of it in the UK. At present, GPs are able to deal more confidently with the chronic sick than the acutely ill. Community-based specialists, working in groups with primary care teams, may be needed to expand provision.

Protocols and guidelines

Attempts are being made everywhere to secure more appropriate delivery of care through the development of guidelines and protocols for clinicians to follow. By means of consensus conferences, New Zealand prepared guidelines for 11 conditions; similar efforts are being made elsewhere.

However, it remains to be seen whether guidelines will be followed by clinicians. In the UK, shared care protocols have proved particularly difficult to formulate and even harder to implement because they require the agreement of GPs as well as specialists.

GP fundholding

In the UK, priorities are also set by GPs who hold budgets. They are said to be better placed to assess demands than district health authorities, but they do not treat enough patients to determine the needs of a whole community and they may make purchasing decisions that could undermine local availability of core services. If priority setting is to proceed in a satisfactory way, co-ordinated action is required to achieve a better balance between the focus on the needs of individual patients and fair use of resources across the community.

Outstanding Issues

Many questions need to be resolved before satisfactory methods of setting priorities can be found. This concluding section sets forth the main ones outstanding.

National direction or local discretion?

In Oregon, priority setting has proceeded on a state-wide basis, but of the other four countries involved in this conference, only the UK has no plans for national direction.

Should priorities be set on a national or local level?

How much direction should come from the central government and how much should be left to local discretion?

What to prioritize, and should there be exclusions?

At present, sufficient information exists only to set priorities within specialties in the form of 'bite-size chunks'. Yet in Oregon an extensive priority list was drawn up which covered the whole spectrum of care, relying on guesswork and judgement to assign many rankings. The Gavleborg Council in Sweden has embarked on a similar course, while in both the Netherlands and New Zealand the intention is to set a basic care package or define a core service. Meanwhile, an inventory or existing services has been taken in New Zealand and an attempt is being made to shift resources among them. By working directly with clinicians to clarify when services should be provided and to whom, it will be possible for policy-makers progressively to identify those services which provide poor net benefit for the cost and to exclude them from publicly funded services, thus freeing up money for other priorities.

Should priorities be set by excluding specific services or merely by shifting resources? Should attempts be made to set priorities across the whole spectrum of care or should efforts be limited to 'bite-size chunks'?

Should the public decide?

Oregon failed to devise a satisfactory method of public consultation and, though surveys made in New Zealand and the Netherlands found support for the development of a basic care package, there was opposition to restriction of services. The Netherlands hopes to overcome this by a three-year public weaning programme, aimed at influential consumer groups.

Should the public be involved in priority setting and what account should be taken of its wishes? If the public is consulted, how should it be done and what attempt, if any, should be made to influence its choices?

Should quality of life be considered?

Federal law in the USA forced Oregon to drop consideration of quality of life issues because they discriminated against
disabled persons. Criticism has also been expressed on the
grounds that they are too subjective to deserve attention.
Yet the use of QALY calculations to determine cost-effectiveness is increasingly being employed elsewhere.

In setting priorities, what account should be taken of the
quality of life produced by treatment?

Does lack of known effects discredit prevention preference?

Priorities everywhere favour prevention and community
care, but few outcome data are available to justify this.
Particular problems could be engendered in the Netherlands, where a strict test of effectiveness is apparently to be
applied, which will rule out all treatments whose worth
cannot be proven. In Sweden, the Gavleborg council offers
a practical alternative, accepting as effective all treatments
for which a wide consensus of worth exits. Yet another
possibility, suggested by a Director of Public Health in the
UK, is to define effectiveness using a method based on
process, such as the extent to which schizophrenics regularly
take the drugs needed for treatment.

Should priorities continue to favour prevention and community care when few outcome data are available to justify
it? If, as seems likely, more outcome data are difficult to
produce, what else can be done to meet the deficiency?

Should age and lifestyle affect priorities?

The age and lifestyle of patients are generally being ruled out as criteria in setting priorities, but they may be taken into consideration by clinicians when assessing outcome. In the UK, age has been a factor in determining access to renal dialysis, and smokers have been denied heart operations, yet it is not always clear that this has been done solely on the basis of an assessment of outcome.

Should age and lifestyle *per se* be adopted as criteria for deciding priorities? If not, what measures can be taken to ensure that they are only applied in an assessment of outcome?

Can protocols work?

Protocols and guidelines have been adopted everywhere in an attempt to secure the delivery of appropriate care, but they have proved difficult to formulate and even harder to implement. This has applied particularly to shared care protocols since they require the agreement of GPs as well as specialists. In New Zealand, boundary guidelines were prepared for 11 conditions by means of consensus conferences involving professionals and lay experts, but no measures have yet been adopted to ensure compliance.

How can purchasers ensure the delivery of appropriate care? If protocols and guidelines are adopted, what can be done to make sure they are implemented?

Can GP fundholding be fair?

In the UK, some GPs themselves hold budgets and set priorities, an arrangement which has enabled them to bring some hospital services closer to the community. However, this arrangement can also create difficulties for district health authorities by restricting their area of influence and threatening the availability of core services. They have also created a two-tier service with hospitals offering preferential treatment to the patients of fundholding GPs.

Should GPs as well as health authorities be allowed to hold budgets and set priorities? If so, what measures can be taken to secure co-ordinated action and avoid a two-tier service?

References and Further Reading

Oregon

Honigsbaum F (1991) *Who shall live? Who shall die?* Oregon's health financing proposals. King's Fund College Papers, London.

Oregon Health Services Commission (Chair: William Gregory) (1991) *Prioritization of health services.* A Report to the Governor and Legislature, Oregon Health Services Commission, Portland, Oregon.

The Netherlands

Government Committee on Choices in Healthcare (Chair: Professor AJ Dunning) (1992) *Choices in healthcare.* Ministry of Health, Welfare and Cultural Affairs, Rijswijk, The Netherlands.

New Zealand

Edgar W (1993) *Core health and disability services – setting priorities in healthcare: the New Zealand experience*. Ministry of Health Wellington

Minister of Health (1991) *The core debate*. Ministry of Health, Wellington.

Minister of Health (1992) *The core debate – review of submissions*. Ministry of Health, Wellington.

National Advisory Committee on Core Health and Disability Support Services (Chair: Sharon Crosbie) (1992) *Core health and disability support services*. Ministry of Health, Wellington.

National Advisory Committee on Core Health and Disability Support Services (1992). *The best of health*. Ministry of Health, Wellington.

National Advisory Committee on Core Health and Disability Support Services (1992). *Consensus development conference reports*. (11 in 1992 and five more to come from conferences held in 1993.) Ministry of Health, Wellington.

National Advisory Committee on Core Health and Disability Support Services (1992). *Seeking consensus*. A discussion document. Ministry of Health, Wellington.

National Advisory Committee on Core Health and Disability Support Services (Chair: Lynette Jones (1993) *Core health and disability support services for 1994/95*. Ministry of Health, Wellington.

National Advisory Committee on Core Health and Disability Support Services (1993). *The best of health 2* Ministry of Health, Wellington.

Sweden

Calltorp J (1989) The 'Swedish model' under pressure – how to maintain equity and develop quality? *Quality Assurance in Health Care*, 1, 13–22.

Calltorp J (1989) *Priority setting and the decision-making process in healthcare. Some post-war characteristics of health policy in Sweden.* Doctoral dissertation at Uppsala University.

Calltorp J (1990) Physician manpower politics in Sweden. *Health Policy*, 15, 105–18.

County Council of Gavleborg (1993) *Setting priorities in healthcare – basic principles.* Gavleborg County Council, Gavleborg.

County Council of Vasterbotten (1993) *Summary of the programme of priorities.* Vasterbotten County Council, Vasterbotten.

The Healthcare and Medical Priorities Commission (Chair: Jerzy Einhorn) (1993) *No easy choices – the difficult priorities of healthcare.* Ministry of Health and Social Affairs, SOU, Stockholm. This is the English version. Priority setting methods in Norway are described on pages 44 of this report.

Holmström S and Calltorp J (1993) *Priority setting in Sweden.* Division of Research and Development, Huddinge Hospital.

Ministry of Health and Social Affairs, statement by Rt. Hon. Bo Konberg (1992) *Priorities in health and social care – committee terms of reference.* Resolution adopted at Cabinet meeting, 30 January 1992. Ministry of Health and Social Affairs, Stockholm.

United Kingdom

Carroll G (1993) Priority setting in purchasing healthcare. In: *Rationing in action*, pp 125–38. British Medical Journal Publishing Group, London.

Ham C, Honigsbaum F and Thompson D (1994) *Priority setting for health gain*. Department of Health, London.

Heginbotham C and Ham C with Cochrane M and Richards J (1992) *Purchasing dilemmas – a special report from the Kings Fund College and Southampton and South West Hampshire Health Authority*. King's Fund College, London.

Hogg S (1993) *Oxfordshire approach to commissioning and priority setting*. Oxfordshire Health Authority, Oxford.

Index